Mohamed BELLALI

Tear gas

AF301155

Mohamed BELLALI

Tear gas

The hidden stakes of medical expertise

This book is a translation from the original published under ISBN 978-620-6-72291-5.

Publisher:
Sciencia Scripts
is a trademark of
Dodo Books Indian Ocean Ltd. and OmniScriptum S.R.L publishing group

120 High Road, East Finchley, London, N2 9ED, United Kingdom
Str. Armeneasca 28/1, office 1, Chisinau MD-2012, Republic of Moldova, Europe
Printed at: see last page
ISBN: 978-620-8-11470-1

CONTENTS

1- INTRODUCTION

Tear gas is a chemical weapon increasingly used by the police to disperse demonstrators during riot control operations. It has the properties of a physical incapacitating agent that rapidly causes short-term temporary disability (1,2).

This weapon is characterised by its low toxicity and the reversibility of its effects if used as recommended. However, certain situations show that it is difficult to control exposure to this gas and that the weapon is not always used correctly, which can cause harm to exposed subjects (3).

Tear gas has been used by the Tunisian police for a number of years, most notably in 2008 during the events in the mining basin, but especially during the riots of December 2010 and January 2011. During the Tunisian revolution in January 2011, a number of demonstrators were exposed to tear gas, some of whom lodged official complaints with the courts. For personal injury experts, exposure to tear gas poses serious problems in terms of proving exposure, establishing the causal link and the medico-legal assessment of the after-effects.

The purpose of this work was to :

- remind us of the harmfulness of this weapon, falsely reputed to be less harmful and less lethal in the short and long term.

- Exhibit the difficulties encountered by the experts during of victims of exposure to tear gas.

2-HISTORY

It is generally accepted that the Maya were the first to use tear gas as a weapon of war to defend themselves against European colonisers in 1605. However, its use really took off during the First World War. France, having discovered the military value of tear gas as early as 1905, used it against the German army in 1914 (4).

In 1925, after the First World War, the Geneva Conventions successively banned these weapons from the law of war. However, their use against civilians remained legal. In 1993, the use of tear gas was banned in armed conflict by an international convention on the prohibition of the development, production, stockpiling and use of chemical weapons and on their destruction (5).

3-CHEMICAL PROPERTIES AND CONCENTRATIONS

There are 3 types of tear gas (1,6-10):

- CN (w-chloroacetophenone) :

It has the molecular formula C_8H_7ClO and a molecular weight of 154.59. It has a melting temperature of around 58-59°C, a boiling point of 244-245°C and a low vapour pressure of $5.4 \times 10-3$ mm Hg at 20°C. CN is practically insoluble in water, although it is freely soluble in ethanol, ether and benzene. CN is a solid, generally disseminated as a particulate aerosol. It is essentially a tear gas. Exposure to a concentration exceeding approximately 1 mg/m^3 induces an abundant flow of tears in less than a minute. The lethal inhalation dose for humans, extrapolated from animal data, is estimated at around 8,500 mg/mn/m3 . CN was developed at the end of the First World War, although it was not used during that war. After the During the First World War, it was widely used by the military and law enforcement agencies until the emergence of other, more powerful and less toxic agents.

- OC or the capsaicin (N- (4-hydroxy-3-methoxybenzyl) - 8methylnontrans 6-enamide):

It occurs naturally in capsicum peppers. Capsaicin has the molecular formula $C_{18}H_{27}NO_3$ and a molecular weight of 305.41. It is solid, off-white in colour, odourless and pungent, with a melting point of around 65°C and a boiling point of 210-220°C. It has a low vapour pressure and is practically insoluble in water, although it is completely soluble in alcohol, ether, chloroform and benzene.

- CS (Chlorobenzylidene Malononitrile) :

It is the agent most commonly used by the police, particularly in France, the United States and Tunisia. It has the molecular formula $C_{10}H_5ClN_2$ and a molecular weight of 188.6. It was discovered in 1928 by British chemists Ben Corson and Roger Stoughton, the name CS being derived from the first letter of both their surnames. It has a cyanocarbon structure. It is a white crystalline solid with a peppery odour, a melting point of around 93°C and a boiling point of 310°C. It has a low vapour pressure and is sparingly soluble in water, although it is soluble in acetone, methylene chloride, ethyl acetate and benzene. CS hydrolyses slightly slowly in water, producing o-chlorobenzaldehyde and malononitrile. Published estimates of lethal doses to humans range from 25,000 to 100,000 mg/min/m^3 . These doses are calculated by extrapolation from results obtained with laboratory animals. The effects of CS are qualitatively quite similar to those of CN, but are more rapid to appear, and occur at lower concentrations. Table 2 provides a brief comparison of the toxicity of the agents.

Table 1: Comparison of the human toxicity of CN, CS and OC (11-13)

	CN	CS	OC
Eye irritation threshold (mg/m3)	1.0	0.004	0.002
Effective concentration-ICt50* (mg/min/m3)	20-50	4-20	-
Estimated lethal dose-ICt50* (in tonnes) (mg/min/m3)	8500-25000	25000-100000	>100000

***ICt50 (average incapacitating concentration)**: The volume of a chemical agent vapour or inhaled aerosol sufficient to incapacitate 50% of exposed, unprotected people.

4-MECHANISMS OF TOXICITY

The mechanism of action of these agents in humans is not fully understood. It is thought that CS and CN act as an alkylating agent possessing the (SN2) group that reacts readily with nucleophilic sites. They cause the inactivation of several nuclear enzymes including lactic dehydrogenase, glutamic dehydrogenase and pyruvic decarboxylase. The inactivation of these metabolic enzyme systems may be linked to exposure-induced tissue damage (14,15).

An additional mechanism of action for tear gas causing irritation and pain may be due to the release of bradykinin (16).

Tear gas targets the TRPA1 receptor, a sensory neuronal receptor that is highly sensitive to irritants. When activated by tear gas, the membrane channels associated with TRPA1 open and allow ca^{2+} ions to enter the cell, causing depolarisation (17). TRPA1 receptors are considered to be the final pathway for inflammatory signalling pathways. The development of TRPA1 antagonists or inhibitors may lead to treatment for tear gas overdose, or even to the use of such antagonists as prophylactics against tear gas (18).

5-USE

Tear gas is used in the form of grenades by police forces to disperse riots. They quickly produce a temporary incapacitating physical irritation or discomfort. They can also be used during police training sessions. The use of tear gas by the police follows precise procedures (19). The grenade can be thrown by hand or with a launcher. A grenade can be thrown by hand up to 15 to 20 metres and 200 metres with a launcher. It can be used individually in the form of a spray or tear gas can for self-defence (2).

6- THE EFFECTS OF TEAR GAS

The effect of tear gas, whatever its type, depends on a number of parameters such as the method of dispersion (gaseous or gel jet), the power of the jet (some bombs can reach up to ten metres), the shape of the dispersion cone (20), whether or not it is thrown directly at the victim, the distance from the victim, the exposed skin surface, the open or confined environment, the means of protection used, effective and rapid decontamination and the victim's history and sensitivity. Under normal conditions of use, symptoms are mainly skin, eye and respiratory irritation, which is significant but transient. However, there are sometimes much more severe symptoms or after-effects (21-23). Deaths have been described and the use of these means of maintaining order has given rise to considerable controversy.

6.1. Short-term effects :

• Ocular effects :

As its name suggests, this gas is tear gas. Its main target is the eyes. It causes intense irritation of exposed mucous membranes, resulting in lacrimation, blepharospasm, conjunctival erythema and periorbital oedema. These symptoms are more severe in victims wearing contact lenses. Permanent eye damage is rare and there have been no cases of blindness in humans as a result of exposure to CS gas or spray. However, elevated intraocular pressure may occur and may precipitate angle-closure glaucoma. Potential longer-term problems include cataract, intravitreal haemorrhage and post-traumatic optic neuropathy

(24-26).

• Respiratory effects:

When tear gas is inhaled, it initially causes nasal congestion and rhinorrhoea. Its burning acid taste reaches the mouth and precedes the tingling effect on the throat. The progression of this gas through the larynx, trachea and bronchi can cause coughing, the production of copious secretions, bronchospasm and laryngospasm. Excessive exposure may result in pulmonary oedema, which may be delayed for up to 24 hours, chemical pneumonitis or congestive heart failure (1,25,27-29). Patients with pre-existing respiratory diseases such as asthma or chronic obstructive pulmonary disease are particularly at risk of more severe reactions and exacerbation of their underlying conditions (17,30,31).

• Dermatological effects:

The skin lesions observed during exposure to tear gas can result either from the flames when the tear gas grenade explodes near the victim, or from contact between the victim's skin and the tear gas grenades thrown by the police, or from the effect of the powder contained in the tear gas canister when it is projected onto the clothing of nearby victims and remains in contact with the victim's skin. On the skin, particularly on the face and eyelids, you may notice irritation such as a burning sensation. and more rarely an erythema without a vesicle. Skin responses to exposure to tear gas are highly variable (32-36).

- **Effects on the digestive tract :**

They are rarely encountered and are rather related to the contamination of food or drink by the gas and not to inhalation. They depend on the degree of irritation of the mucous membranes and result in the appearance of symptoms such as nausea, vomiting, lack of appetite, diarrhoea and abdominal pain (8,9,23,31).

6.2 Long-term effects :

Tear gas causes temporary clinical symptoms which disappear a few minutes or even a few hours after exposure. More rarely, the inhalation of tear gas and in particular conditions of location and concentration of inhaled gas can cause long-term symptoms, particularly respiratory: this is **the Reactive Airways Dysfunction Syndrome (RADS) or Brooks syndrome**. This syndrome poses a twofold problem for medical experts: the first is diagnostic and the second concerns imputability to exposure to tear gas. RADS will be discussed in more detail later.

7-TEAR GAS AND DEATH

Our review of the literature showed no data concerning cases of death caused by inhalation of tear gas. However, there are rare cases of death caused by tear gas canisters. This projectile can behave like a blunt object, causing serious trauma and death through its kinetic energy.Worldwide, fatal injuries caused by tear gas canisters are not exclusively head injuries. Trauma to the chest and neck can be fatal (37-40). Tear gas can also cause serious but non-fatal trauma (cranial, facial, thoracic, etc.) likely to leave after-effects for the victims (41). In this situation, the medical expert will be called upon to assess the after-effects and set the level of disability.

8-TREATMENT

In cases of exposure to tear gas, the affected individuals should be removed as quickly as possible from the area where the spray was used. They should then be exposed to fresh air, which will speed up eye decontamination. In cases where victims are showing severe respiratory symptoms, normobaric oxygen therapy is indicated. Contaminated clothing should be removed and placed in a plastic bag. The eyes should be washed as quickly as possible with a saline solution or cool water to reduce the burning sensation and facilitate elimination of the active ingredient. This treatment also helps to avoid the complications mentioned above (42,43). If contact lenses are worn, they should be removed quickly and decontaminated before reuse. If the pain persists and the patient remains unable to open his eyes, it is advisable to irrigate the palpebral cul-de-sac, as the tear gas tends to collect there and remain trapped. In the event of ocular inflammation, non-steroidal anti-inflammatory drugs or corticosteroids may be used. The face, and in particular the eyelids, should be decontaminated with a mild soap, avoiding rubbing and sponging to avoid facilitating the penetration of the toxic substance, which is highly lipophilic (17,43). Victims should wash their hands to avoid recontaminating their eyes. Medical staff must use gloves to avoid transferring contamination to themselves and to patients (27,44,45).

9- REACTIVE AIRWAY DYSFUNCTION SYNDROME

9.1. Definition:

Brooks syndrome or **Reactive Airways Dysfunction Syndrome (RADS)** was first described in 1985 by Brooks and defined as the onset of symptoms suggestive of asthma within 24 hours of exposure to a gas, vapour or fume with irritant properties in high concentration. These symptoms are accompanied by bronchial obstruction and/or non-specific bronchial hyperresponsiveness (46,47). It refers to asthma, due to a **single** acute inhalation of an irritant gas, which may even in the absence of an initial transient bronchospasm evolve over months or years. Tear gas is one of the irritants that can cause this syndrome.

9.2. Pathophysiology :

In RADS, the acute, immediate symptoms are certainly due to inflammation of the airways. Massive exposure leads to massive alteration and destruction of the bronchial epithelium, followed by direct activation of non-adrenergic, non-cholinergic inflammation pathways via anoxic reflexes. Non-specific activation of macrophages and degranulation of mast cells may also occur, with the release of chemotactic and toxic mediators. Secondary recruitment of inflammatory cells to the lesion then accentuates and sustains the inflammatory response (48). Damage to the epithelium appears to be the initial key factor: it alters the intrinsic function of epithelial cells and leads to the release of inflammatory mediators by these cells, resulting in changes in microvascular permeability and increased mucus secretion (49).

However, the reason why asthma develops in certain individuals is unclear. Several hypotheses have been put forward to explain the persistence of bronchial hyperresponsiveness, including :

➢ The threshold of irritation receptors in the airways is altered as a result of re-epithelialisation and re-innervation of the airways.
➢ Increased permeability in the airway walls following damage to the bronchial mucosa, giving easier access to irritation receptors for inhaled substances.
➢ The very prolonged alteration in the reactivity of the smooth muscle following the massive release of mediators during the inhalation accident and the inflammatory reaction.
➢ Persistent bronchial inflammation.

9.3. Results of bronchial biopsies :

Biopsies very regularly show :

- lesions of the respiratory epithelium, with more or less massive destruction.

- pseudo-thickening of the basement membrane which, when studied ultrastructurally, appears to be due to sub-epithelial fibrosis with accumulation of collagen fibres, the integrity of the basement membrane being preserved.

- the bronchial submucosa is the site of an inflammatory reaction that is usually moderate, mainly mononuclear, and above all non-specific, with no eosinophilic infiltrate.

9.4. General characteristics :

Victims are more likely to be men aged between 30 and 40. Smoking does not appear to play a significant role. Atopy is not more common among sufferers. Exposure to the toxic substance generally lasts from a few minutes to 12 hours (50).

9.5. Positive diagnosis :

Diagnosis is based on the demonstration of an obstructive ventilatory disorder on functional respiratory testing (FRT), spontaneously or after a bronchial provocation test with methacoline in a previously symptom-free subject, following a single exposure to an irritant agent (gas, smoke, etc.). Obstructive ventilatory disorder is detected by functional respiratory investigation (FRI):

• A lower forced expiratory volume in one second (FEV1) of less than 80% of the theoretical value

• A Tiffeneau coefficient (FEV1/CV) is also lowered.

9.6. The clinical state at a distance from the accident :

RADS is characterised by the persistence of asthma attacks with bronchial hyperresponsiveness after the initial accident. The frequency and severity of the attacks may intensify. Between attacks, there is often an obstructive syndrome that is incompletely reversible under adrenergic therapy, which distinguishes the syndrome from benign allergic asthma. The intensity of exposure is the main factor in the onset and severity of RADS. All in all, the course of the disease can be summarised as follows: half the patients progress towards a cure, a quarter remain stable and a quarter suffer a worsening of their condition. The importance of the initial clinical signs and perhaps the early presence of an obstructive syndrome and bronchial hyperresponsiveness are negative factors. There is no evidence that early corticosteroid therapy can prevent the development of RADS (50-53).

10- SPECIAL FEATURES OF FORENSIC EXAMINATION OF EXPOSURE VICTIMS

10.1. Tear gas and imputability :

In medico-legal terms, imputability is the study of the relationship between the trauma, the initial injuries and the after-effects observed. It is not always easy to establish the causal link, particularly when there is a previous pathological condition or when several events have contributed, in varying proportions of responsibility, to the genesis of the injury.

The establishment of an imputability link is based on the study of a set of so-called "imputability" criteria. These criteria, initially described by Maurice Müller and Cordonnier in 1925 and then revised by Simonien (54,55), are broadly seven in number:

• **Reality of the trauma:** For the imputability of the damage to be recognised in relation to an event (trauma), the latter must be real and proven.

• **Intensity:** In order to cause damage, a trauma must be sufficiently intense to generate disorders. However, there are exceptions to this criterion, insofar as a trauma, without being serious and intense, can lead to secondary disorders.

• **Concordance of site:** In principle, damage must appear in the region of the body where the trauma occurred. This notion may be lacking for certain types of endocrine disruption caused by traumatic stress.

• **Logical delay between trauma and damage:** This criterion is in fact difficult to standardise and remains variable depending on the damage. For example, some disorders may develop early in the aftermath of a trauma, while others may develop much later, sometimes taking years to appear. The length of this delay does not rule out imputability, but rather attenuates it. Some injuries require a longer delay (e.g. necrosis of the femoral head, post-traumatic epilepsy).

• **Continuity of symptoms:** In general, symptoms and residual functional discomfort should evolve continuously between the initial trauma and the final state. For some injuries, however, this rule may not apply (e.g. the appearance of epilepsy years after a head injury).

• **Pathogenic plausibility:** A disorder can only be recognised as a sequelae attributable to a trauma if there is a scientifically accepted mechanism proving that the disorder may result from the trauma.

• **Absence of a prior condition:** Damage can only be attributed to a traumatic event if there is no prior pathological condition. The existence of the latter would make the process part of an interaction mechanism (aggravation, triggering, etc.) between the 2 events rather than an initial genesis.

In order to attribute exposure to RADS, a set of criteria defined by Brooks must be present. There are 8 criteria (23):

➢ No previous respiratory complaints ;

➢ Initial onset of respiratory problems after a single exposure to bronchial irritants ;

➢ Exposure to high concentrations of irritating gases, vapours, aerosols, fumes and dusts;

➢ Respiratory problems appear within 24 hours of exposure and persist for at least three months;

➢ Asthma-like symptoms with the urge to cough, attacks of respiratory discomfort or dyspnoea on exertion, presence of sibilant rales on clinical examination;

➢ Possible obstructive ventilatory disorder on EFR;

➢ Positive metacholine test ;

➢ Exclusion of other bronchopulmonary diseases ;

In our series, two of the 27 victims of exposure to tear gas had retained a RADS. These victims had validated the 8 imputability criteria.

The imputability of RADS to tear gas inhalation must be based on the chronology and circumstances of exposure. The appearance of symptoms within 24 hours is a major diagnostic criterion, but here again, its application must be measured: the onset of disorders may be slightly delayed, exceeding 24 hours (56). Several authors have already discussed the relevance of the first criterion, the absence of previous respiratory complaints. In fact, the victim's condition may have worsened. For example, the diagnosis of RADS was accepted in the case of a former asthmatic exposed to nitrous oxide during the derailment of a train in Louisiana in 1995: this patient was asymptomatic and had not been taking any treatment for many years (56). The existence of a history of allergic asthma or COPD in the victims should not lead to a rejection of the diagnosis. In our series, the diagnosis of RADS was retained in two other victims despite the presence of a history of respiratory pathology.

10.2. Tear gas and previous condition :

➤ Definition:

According to Professor Fagnart (57), the anterior state is an abnormal situation in the physiology, anatomy or psyche of the individual, creating either an established pathology or a latent state (itself already pathological but not yet having clinical manifestations) (58).

It is also defined as the victim's condition prior to t h e accident (59).

It can also be defined as "an injury report, i.e. a medical report listing the pathologies from which a person was suffering or had suffered prior to the accident in question". Medical doctrine also considers that the antecedent condition "consists of all the antecedents likely to be involved in the pathological process following the accident.

➤ Difficulties of the appraisal in relation to the previous condition :

Several difficulties may co-exist in the face of a previous condition such as:

• Recognition of the previous state, definition of its limits and its painful and functional repercussions before the trauma occurred.
• Lack of parallelism between the information provided, particularly by imaging, and the functional impact of the previous pathology,

• The difficulty of obtaining reliable information about this prior condition from the injured person, who may have an interest in masking it or denying its consequences.

• Difficulty in obtaining medical documents containing information about the patient's previous condition, such as a hospital report or a certificate from the attending physician.

➤ **How do you find the previous state?**

The search for the previous state by the medical expert must be carried out throughout all the stages of the expert assessment

-The medical history: For each antecedent, it will be necessary to be precise about the dates and periods of hospitalisation, time off work, etc. However, it must be recognised that the examining doctor can only seek information relating to a previous condition by Based on what the patient is willing to reveal and provide as documents in compliance with medical confidentiality.

-Clinical examination: This is used to identify clinical signs associated with a particular pathology and to bring up forgotten antecedents with the patient (e.g. laparotomy scars or bone deformities).

-Possible recourse to specialist advice: This involves recourse to a qualified health professional (specialist doctor, speech therapist, psychologist, occupational therapist, prosthetist) to give an opinion or useful information on the condition. The doctor must remain in control of the questions he asks. It is not up to the consultant to take the place of the expert.

-Communication of documents relating to the previous condition: This is easy if the "victim" is cooperative. They are the owners of the medical information concerning them. More specifically, this includes operating reports, hospital reports, anatomopathological results and medical certificates. The expert has no direct power to obtain the documents he needs. In criminal cases, he may do so through the examining magistrate or the police authority that requested it.

➢ **Influence of trauma o n   previous state :**

Trauma can influence the previous state. It can :

• **Reveal:** Revelation is the action of making known what was unknown (previous state or predisposition). This does not imply any obvious prior pathology. The trauma is unrelated to this condition and only played a revealing role. The reason for this revelation may be a radiological examination, a biological examination or the physical examination carried out by the doctor(60-62).

• **Triggering:** Triggering is the phenomenon that causes disorders to appear that did not previously exist. Triggering excludes any proven prior pathology. "We can only trigger what was not previously triggered" (61). Triggering presupposes, by definition, that the trauma causes the appearance of a disorder which did not previously exist and which, without this event, would not have existed in the same circumstances. This disorder may be favoured by the victim's predisposition or basic personality, but before the trauma, the victim was not suffering from any pathology.

• **Decompensate:** Prior to the trauma, a clinically proven pathological condition existed but was compensated for either naturally or by treatment. The trauma may lead to a temporary decompensation of the previous condition which was silent and justify a TIW and a quantum doloris or give rise to a lasting decompensation which will also justify the attribution of a PPI.

- **Aggravation:** In reality, we can only talk about aggravation if there is a synergy between the previous condition and the new disability. This synergy will exist when the accident affects the function that was already impaired by the proven previous condition. On the other hand, if there is a new injury affecting a function other than that affected by the proven previous condition, there is a a simple juxtaposition of injuries. The new disability is totally independent of the previous proven condition.

Aggravation consists of going from a level of discomfort C1 to a level of discomfort C2 with $C2 \geq C1$ (for example, from moderate discomfort to severe discomfort). The rate of permanent partial disability (PPD) is then calculated using the Gabrieli formula as a guide:

Disability resulting f r o m a second trauma :

C1-C2 / C1

Where **C1**= Remaining capacity from a previous trauma.

C2= Remaining capacity of a current trauma.

- **Accentuate /Accelerate:** Acceleration refers to the effect of the trauma on a proven and evolving previous state. The previous state, independently of the trauma, should have led to the state observed at the time of the trauma. However, the evolutionary process was accelerated by the trauma.

Confirmation of acceleration is difficult to establish. It is based essentially on the presence in the subject, prior to the trauma, of a pathology of the progressive type in the sense of an ineluctable aggravation leading to a serious condition, or even death, and on the fact that longevity in such cases has been shortened.

• **Neutral:** The trauma is unrelated to the previous condition. The patient tries to attribute everything to the trauma in order to increase t h e rate of PPI. The expert does not find in In general, it is difficult to rule out any link between the trauma and the previous condition.

10.3. Tear gas and associated trauma:

Although there is no apparent interaction between exposure to tear gas and trauma, a sufficiently violent trauma can render the victim immobile, which can prolong the duration of the victim's exposure to the gas. On the other hand, inhalation of the gas neutralises the victim and exposes him or her to attack by the police.

11- THE DIFFICULTIES OF ASSESSING VICTIMS OF EXPOSURE TO TEAR GAS

11.1. In relation to the quality of the initial medical certificate :

The initial medical certificate (IMC) is the cornerstone of the assessment of bodily injury: it is the evidence of the reality of the trauma on which the expert doctor bases his assessment of the injury suffered by the victim. As a result, a good-quality IMC facilitates the expert's task of determining the after-effects and determining whether the after-effects are attributable to the traumatic event. An initial quality medical certificate must first be dated the day it is drawn up and must include the identity of the doctor (surname, first name, position, address), the identity of the patient and, in the event of a requisition, the requesting authority. This document must also mention, in the conditional, the facts alleged by the person, with the date and type of violence suffered. The doctor, without questioning his patient's statements, cannot attest to a situation that he has not witnessed directly. The length of time between the alleged events and the medical examination may be noted on the certificate. The practitioner will take care to indicate only the person's history that may be linked to the violence reported. The certificate must also stipulate the documents provided by the patient, in particular any additional examinations carried out and submitted and any days spent in hospital. The functional signs and complaints described by the patient should be recorded. This is followed by the medical examination, with an indication of the place, date and time, and a description of the injuries that appear to be traumatic. This description is important and is well codified. The description must be exact and precise, indicating the type, colour, shape, size (width, length, depth) and location in relation to obvious anatomical landmarks for each lesion observed. The terms used must be appropriate (63,64). If no lesion is visible on clinical examination, this should be stated. Negative findings are as important as positive ones. The patient may report pain with no visible skin lesion. It will be necessary to describe whether there is any muscle contracture (particularly in the cervical, dorsal or lumbar spine), or oedema indicating a sprain mechanism, for example. In all cases, the description of the injury should be supplemented by a search for functional disability or impotence, describing it in terms of substance and intensity. The presence or absence of discomfort in dressing, walking, grasping, or getting up from a chair or examination table may be noted (64).

11.2. In connection with the simulation of victims :

The simulation behaviour of these victims can be explained by the very high stakes involved in this expertise, which is to be included on the list of those wounded in the revolution. In this situation, the medical expert, in addition to his clinical skills, must have knowledge of psychopathology and behaviour in order to be able to detect a simulating victim (65-68).

The Diagnostic and Statistical Manual of Mental Disorders drawn up by the American Psychiatric Association **(DSM-V)** (69) defines malingering as "the intentional production of inauthentic or grossly exaggerated physical or psychological symptoms". motivated by external incentives such as avoiding military obligations, avoiding work, obtaining financial compensation, avoiding legal proceedings or obtaining drugs". The DSM-V considers that malingering should be strongly suspected in the presence of one or more of the following manifestations:

1. existence of a medico-legal context ;

2. significant discrepancy between the suffering or disability reported by the subject and the objective results of the examination ;

3. lack of cooperation during diagnostic assessment and failure to comply with prescribed medical treatment ;

4. existence of an antisocial personality.

Simulation is at the origin of a whole series of behaviours that must however be taken into account, which are of 3 types:

- **Pure simulation"**, in which the subject invents from scratch a set of symptoms or deficits that do not exist.

- **Exaggeration of** existing disorders or oversimulation (deliberate exaggeration of a real condition). In this fairly frequent type of behaviour, the simulator exploits and amplifies a pre-existing morbid disorder.

- **Fixation of** disorders that have actually disappeared. In this case, the subject will persevere in his attitude of simulation.

The desire to simulate does not always stem from an interest in obtaining financial compensation, but may also be based on the simulator's need to be recognised as a victim. In dealing with the traumatic event and its consequences, those around them can play a major role in the adoption of certain simulation behaviours. Children are a special case in this respect. People close to a child (particularly parents) play a major role in the adoption of malingering behaviour.

In terms of the medico-legal principles guiding the assessment of heads of loss, the discussion is limited by two boundaries (67) :

- massive **under-assessment**, by underestimating the authenticity and seriousness of the picture and suffering, especially in the case of psychological complaints.

- **an over-evaluation**, simply recording the subject's grievances without being able to analyse them.

In the case of victims with simulated organic sequelae, questioning, clinical examination and additional tests enable the expert doctor to detect these cases easily. However, in the case of simulated neuropsychological sequelae, the diagnosis becomes more delicate and requires, in addition to the usual examinations, the following:

- scales to assess fascist potential (F scale), Structured Interview of Reported Symptoms (SIRS) and the Structured Inventory of Malingered Symptomatology (SIMS).

- simulation cues such as latency (deliberately producing incorrect responses would require longer information processing than producing correct responses), cues such as the types of errors produced, the presence or absence of perseveration and in the child by the lack of sophistication and inconsistent performance shown and influence (the coaching) detected by clinical observation of parent-child interactions. However, all these methods are controversial in terms of effectiveness and validity (66,68).

The expert's role is to be a good listener, using a benevolent, professional and neutral approach, in order to understand the expert's difficulties as well as possible. The climate of listening and empathy created by the expert is a fundamental criterion that must enable the person undergoing the expertise to express his suffering authentically: the latter will feel less need to simulate in order to ensure that he is recognised as a victim (65). Furthermore, the expert must not, in an attempt to defuse possible malingering, become a malingerer himself by trying to show himself to be biased and overly favourable a priori. The expert's only role is to enlighten the judge and he has no decision-making power: this is what characterises his neutrality, which must be maintained, even when we want to establish a climate of trust (66).

11.3. In connection with the victims :

In Tunisia, an elderly person within the meaning of article 1 of law no. 94-114 of 31/10/1994, relating to the protection of the elderly, is anyone over the age of 60. From a biological point of view, ageing is the product of the accumulation of a vast array of molecular and cellular damage over time. This leads to a progressive deterioration in physical and mental capacities, an increased risk of disease and, finally, death. Ageing starts early, but its The effects are only perceptible from the age of 50 onwards, and are essentially characterised by a reduction in the individual's functional reserves, leading to increasing difficulty in adapting to new situations and developing strategies, in other words, resisting and coping.

Ageing has a phenotypic impact on a number of functions, such as muscle mass, bone mass, heart function, liver function and kidney function. Ageing also affects respiratory function: Respiratory ageing is somewhat unusual in that it is the consequence of a stiffening of the thoracic cage and also of sarcopenia, which affects the muscles of the thoracic cage. With advancing age, there is a reversal of air flow and vascular flow. Younger people breathe and ventilate at the base of the body, where haematosis occurs. With age, ventilation in the apices becomes more important as a result of impaired diaphragmatic mechanics. The best-ventilated areas are less well perfused, leading to hypoxaemia and a reduction in alveolar surface area. The combination of cardiac and pulmonary ageing contributes to the progressive onset of exercise-induced deconditioning. This physiological reduction in respiratory capacity has posed a problem for experts when assessing respiratory sequelae in victims of exposure to tear gas (70).

Forensic analysis of the elderly person cannot therefore ignore their particular life trajectory, which is studded with events and marked by the physiological phenomenon of ageing, which collides with the hazards of life (71). What is essential when assessing the person The search for a previous condition in the elderly is more difficult than in middle-aged people. Searching for a previous condition in an elderly person is more difficult than in a middle-aged person, because this condition is deliberately or inadvertently concealed by those around them or by the person themselves, partly because they do not want to see their loved ones grow old, and partly because they have simply forgotten a pathological past that has been relegated to the background. The expert doctor cannot carry out a post-traumatic assessment without also having a precise and complete description of the elements of autonomy, by placing this person in his or her social fabric, in his or her aids such as they were exactly before the event to manage themselves. The role of the medical expert is to describe only those after-effects that are directly and definitely related to the injuries. In addition to the after-effects, the accident may also lead to a social imbalance, sometimes requiring the use of aids, sometimes obliging the patient to change her lifestyle, which may even involve a change of location. The role of the medical expert is to describe this change in situation, specifying the respective roles of the accident, the patient's previous condition and any family or friends (70).

When carrying out a medical examination of an elderly person, the expert must not forget three key elements to be studied:

• The functional impact of the accident,

• The victim's previous condition,

• The impact on the victim's autonomy.

12-CONCLUSION

Tear gas is a chemical weapon increasingly used by the police to disperse demonstrators during riot control operations. It has the properties of a physical incapacitating agent that rapidly causes short-term temporary disability. This weapon is characterised by its low toxicity and the reversibility of its effects if used as recommended. This gas can cause harm to exposed subjects. During the Tunisian revolution in January 2011, a number of demonstrators were exposed to tear gas, some of whom have lodged official complaints with the courts.For personal injury experts, exposure to tear gas poses serious problems in terms of proving exposure, establishing the causal link and the medico-legal assessment of the after-effects. Recognition of the causal link between exposure to tear gas and the sequelae found is based on verification of the criteria of imputability, which are: the reality of the exposure, the reality of the condition through its diagnosis, the concordance of the seat between exposure and the sequellary disorder, as well as the time of onset of this disorder, the chronological sequence of symptoms since the exposure, the absence of a previous condition and a cause unrelated to the exposure. It is sometimes difficult to verify these criteria because of the victim's previous condition, the quality of the initial medical certificate, the simulation of victims and the determination of after-effects in elderly people.

REFERENCES

1. C. Bismuth. CHEMICAL WEAPONS Description and toxic risks. Réanimation Urgences. 1993;2(6):625-33.

2. Baert A, V. Danel. Chemical weapons. EMC - Toxicol Pathol. 2004;1:117-23.

3. Amnesty International: Israel and the Occupied Territories: The Misuse of Tear Gas by Israeli Army Personnel in the Israeli Occupied Territories, London, 1 June 1988.

4. Lion O. Des armes maudites pour les sales guerres ? l'emploi des armes chimiques dans les conflits asymétriques. Stratégique. 2009;1:491-531.

5. CONVENTION ON THE PROHIBITION OF THE DEVELOPMENT, PRODUCTION, STOCKPILING AND USE OF CHEMICAL WEAPONS AND ON THEIR DESTRUCTION. 2005:1-169.

6. Dibenz B, Blain PG. Tear Gases and Irritant Incapacitants. Toxical Rev. 2003;22(2):103-10.

7. HEALTH ASPECTS OF CHEMICAL AND BIOLOGICAL WEAPONS
Report of a WHO Group of Consultants. 1969:1-132.

8. Zucchetti M, Torino P. Environmental and human damage caused by CS tear gas. TCIMAIL. 2011;1-6.

9. Schep LJ, Slaughter RJ, Mcbride DI. Riot control agents: the tear gases CN , CS and OC - a medical review. J R Army Med Corps.

2013;59:1-6.

10. Malhotra RC, Kumar P. Chemistry and Toxicity of Tear Gases. Def Sci J. 1987;37(2):281-96.

11. Carron PN, Yersin B. Management of the effects of exposure to tear gas.

BMJ. 2009;338:b2283.

12. Olajos EJ, Salem H. Riot control agents: pharmacology, toxicology, biochemistry andchemistry. J Appl Toxicol. 2001;21:355-91.

13. Steffee CH, Lantz PE, Flannagan LM, et al. Oleoresin capsicum (pepper) spray and "in-custody deaths". Am J Forensic Med Pathol. 1995;16:185-92.

14. Sanford JP. Medical aspects of riot control (harassing) agents. Annu Rev Med. 1976;27:421-9.

15. Worthington E, Nee PA. CS exposure-clinical effects and management.

J Accid Emerg Med. 1999;16:168-70.

16. Cucinell SA, Swentzel KC, Biskup R, et al. Biochemical interactions and metabolic fate of riot control agents. Fed Proc. 1971;30:86-91.

17. E. FONTAN. Pepper sprays replace tear gas for private individuals. J Med Leg Droit Med. 2007;50:279-85.

18. Brône B, Peeters PJ, Marrannes R, Mercken M, Nuydens R, Meert

T, et al. Tear gasses CN , CR , and CS are potent activators of the human TRPA1 receptor. Toxicol Appl Pharmacol. 2008;231:150-6.

19. BL.Danto .Medical problems and criteria regarding the use oftear gas by police. Am J Forensic Med Pathol. 1987;8:317-22.

20. VW.Sidel, RM.Goldwyn. Chemical and biological weapons:a primer.
M.D. N Engl J Med. 1966;274:21-27.

21. J.M.Sapori. Chemical weapons for law enforcement. In: Society of Clinical Toxicology. 2012. p. 1-13.

22. P.J.Anderson. Acute effects of the potent lacrimator o-chlorobenzylidene malononitrile (CS) tear gas. Hum Exp Toxicol. 1996;15:461-5.

23. Dimitroglou Y, Rachiotis G, Hadjichristodoulou C. Exposure to the Riot Control Agent CS and Potential Health Effects: A Systematic Review of the Evidence. Int J Environ Res Public Heal. 2015;12:1397-411.

24. Hoffmann DH. EYE BURNS CAUSED BY TEAR GAS. Brit J Ophthal. 2000;51:265-8.

25. Horton DK, Berkowitz Z, Kaye WE. Secondary Contamination of ED Personnel From Hazardous Materials Events, 1995-2001. Am J Emerg Med. 2003;21:199-204.

26. Yih JP. CS gas injury to the eye [editorial]. BMJ. 1995;311:276.

27. Worthington E, Nee PA. CS exposure-clinical effects and management. J Accid Emerg Med. 1999;16:168-70.

28. Arbak P, Ba EG, Kumbasar ÖO, Ülger F, Zeki KJJ, Evyapan F. Long Term Effects of Tear Gases on Respiratory System: Analysis of 93 Cases. Sci World J. 2014;5-9.

29. Park S, Jolla L. Toxic Effects of Tear Gas on an Infant Following Prolonged Exposure. amer J dis cild. 2015;123:245-6.

30. Acute pulmonary effects from o-chlorobenzylidenemalonitrile "tear gas": A unique exposure outcome unmasked by strenuous exercise after a military training event. Mil Med. 2002;167:136-9.

31. Blain PG. Human Incapacitants [Internet]. First Edit. CLINICAL NEUROTOXICOLOGY: Syndromes, Substances, Environments. 2016:660-673

32. Ro YS, Lee CW. Tear Gas Dermatitis Allergic ContactSensitization due to CS.   int J Dermatol. 1991;30(8):576-7.

33. Agrawal Y, Thornton D, Phipps A. CS gas - Completely safe? A burn case report and literature review. BURNS. 2009;35:895-7.

34. John S, Thomas S. Unintended cutaneous reactions to CS spray. Contact Dermatitis. 2005;53:9-13.

35. S.Sommer, SM.Wilkinson. Exposure-pattern dermatitis due to CS gas.

Contact Dermatitis. 1999;40:46-7.

36. Parneix-Spake A, Al. AT et. Severe Cutaneous Reaction to Self-Defense Sprays. Arch Dermatol. 1993;129:913.

37. Clarot F, Vaz E. Lethal head injury due to tear-gas cartridge

gunshots. Forensic Sci Int. 2003;137:45-51.

38. Toprak S, Ersoy G, Hart J, Clevestig P. The pathology of lethal exposure to the Riot Control Agents: Towards a forensics-based methodology for determining misuse. J Forensic Leg Med. 2016;29:36-42.

39. Schmidt U, Schöning R, Krause D, Mckeon P. Death from "non-lethal" firearm. Lancet. 1998;352:1941-2.

40. Rothschild MA, Vendura K. Fatal neck injuries caused by blank cartridges. Forensic Sci Int. 1999;101:151-9.

41. S.Corbacioglu et al. Rare and Severe Maxillofacial Injury Due to Tear Gas Capsules: Report of Three Cases. J Forensic Sci. 2016;61(2):551-4.

42. Karagama YG, Newton JR, Newbegin CJR. Short-term and long-term physical effects of exposure to CS spray. J R Soc Med. 2003;24:7-9.

43. B.Viala, Blomet J. PREVENTION OF CS "TEAR GAS" EYE AND SKIN EFFECTS AND ACTIVE DECONTAMINATION WITH DIPHOTERINE: PRELIMINARY STUDIES IN 5 FRENCH GENDARMES. J Emerg Med. 2005;29(1):5-8.

44. Sivathasan N. Educating on CS or " tear gas ." Emerg Med J. 2010;27:881-3.

45. Rappert B. Health and safety in policing: lessons from the regulation of CS sprays in the UK. Soc Sci Med. 2003;56:1269-78.

46. Lemière C. Syndrome d ' irritation bronchique. Rev Fr Allergol

Immunol. 2001;41:294-300.

47. Hill, A.R.; Silverberg, N.B.; Mayorga, D.; Baldwin, H.E. Medical hazards of the tear gas CS. A case of persistent, multisystem, hypersensitivity reaction and review of the literature. Medicine (Baltimore). 2000;79,234-240.

48. HU H, D C. Reactive airways dysfunction after exposure to teargas. Lancet. 1992;339:1535.

49. Hout.J, White.W. o-Chlorobenzylidene Malononitrile (CS Riot Control Agent) Associated Acute Respiratory Illnesses in a U. S. Army Basic Combat Training Cohort. Mil Med. 2014;179:793-9.

50. N R. Brooks syndrome. Irritant-induced asthma. Doc pour le médecin du Travail. 2000;82:153-9.

51. Brooks SM, Weiss MA, Bernstein IL. Reactive Airways Dysfunction Syndrome (RADS). Chest [Internet]. 1985;88(3):376-84.

52. Deschamps D, Gervais P, Questel F. Le syndrome de dysfonction reactive des voies aériennes et les asthmes toxiques. Rev Fr Allergo Immuno Clin. 1996;36(8):960-6.

53. Roth VS, Franzblau A. RADS after exposure to a riot-control agent: A case report.J Occup Environ Med. 1996;38,863-865.

54. Vayre P, Planquelle D, Fabre H. Le lien de causalité en matière de responsabilité médicale. Médecine & Droit. 2005 ; 05 :78-84.

55. Roberge D. Guide de l'expert. 1st edition. Québec: Direction de la vigie; 2004.

56. Testud F. Brooks syndrome: more flexibility in the application of

diagnostic criteria. REV PNEUMOL CLIN. 2004;60:154-7.

57. Lucas P, Rixhon E. Predispositions and prior condition. In: Fagnart JL, ed. Nouvelles approches des préjudices corporels - Évolution ! Revolution? Resolutions... . Liège : Jeune barreau; 2009.p.35.

58. Fight I. Prior condition of the victim, real questions or false debates? In: De Boe Cet al, dir. Droit médical et dommages corporels - État des lieux et perspectives. Limal : Anthemis ; 2014.p.195.

59. RIJCKMANS M. Essai d'une approche concrète de la notion d'état antérieur [Thesis]. Evaluation du dommage corporel: Brussels; 1995. 204 p.

60. Fagnart JL. La causalité et la réceptivité de la victime [Online]. THELIUS law firm [cited 27/04/2015].

61. Vayre P. Incidences de l'état antérieur en expertise médico-légale. J Chir. 1997;134:86-88.

62. Roberge D. Guide de l'expert. 1st edition. Québec: Direction de la vigie;2004.

63. Ferrant O, Sec I. Le certificat médical initial. J Eur des Urgences Réanimation. Elsevier Masson SAS; 2016;24(2):101-4.

64. Europ J, Autorit H, Sas EM. Synthesis of the recommendations of GOOD PRACTICE . Initial medical certificate concerning a victim of violence. J Eur des Urgences Réanimation. 2012;24:105-13.

65. Zagury D. " The zero and the infinite". About the most
controversial situations in forensic science. Rev Fr Dommage Corp.
2012;2:101-5.

66. Blavier A. Simulation behaviour in the context
Expertise in particular: towards a better understanding of the
victimology process. Evol Psychiatr. 2011;76(2):345-59.

67. Mol J De, Staquet P. La surenchère dans l'expertise psychiatrique.
Rev Fr Dommage Corp. 2008;1:69-84.

68. Roure LP. Lying and simulation: psychiatric and criminological
aspects of sincerity. Paris: Masson; 1996.

69. Battle DE. Cautionary Statement for Forensic Use of DSM-5. In:
Diagnostic and Statistical Manual of Mental Disorders, 5th Edition.
American Psychiatric Publishing, Inc; 2013. p. 191-2.

70. Rodat O, Ment RCLÉ. Expertise médico-légale du sujet âgé ou
comment éviter la tentation de " l'âgisme ". Rev Fr Dommage Corp.
2005;3:19-30.

71. Ruby PY. Bilan d'un état fragile lors de l'expertise de la personne
âgée Proposition d'une grille d'évaluation. Rev Fr Dommage Corp.
2005;3:51-3.

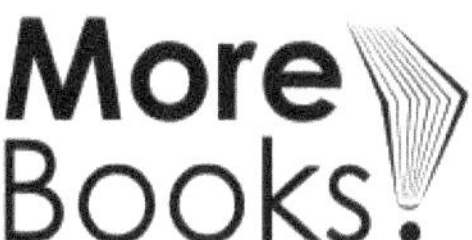

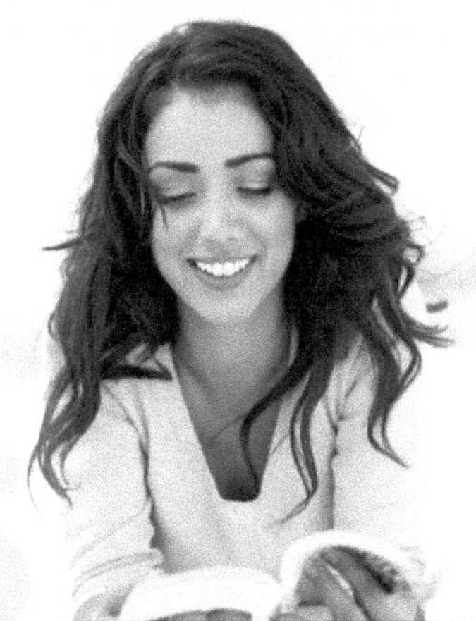

I want morebooks!

Buy your books fast and straightforward online - at one of world's fastest growing online book stores! Environmentally sound due to Print-on-Demand technologies.

Buy your books online at
www.morebooks.shop

Kaufen Sie Ihre Bücher schnell und unkompliziert online – auf einer der am schnellsten wachsenden Buchhandelsplattformen weltweit! Dank Print-On-Demand umwelt- und ressourcenschonend produziert.

Bücher schneller online kaufen
www.morebooks.shop

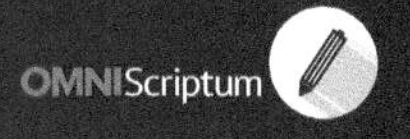

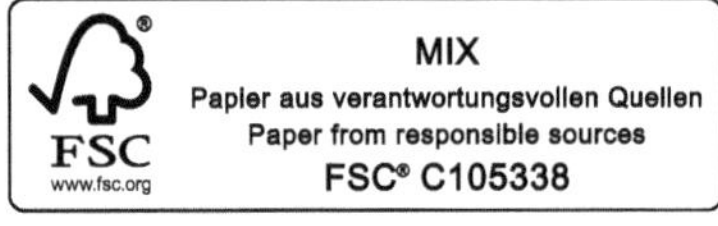